SARAH'S JOURNEY:

"A TALE OF RESILIENCE AND SELF-DISCOVERY"

By

DR FAITH STONES

Table of Contents

Introduction

In a world where societal pressures and self-doubt often overshadow the journey towards self-acceptance and holistic well-being, "Sarah's Journey: A Tale of Resilience and Self-Discovery" serves as a guiding light, illuminating the transformative power of determination, self-compassion, and the unwavering commitment to embracing a lifestyle that thrives on the abundance of inner strength and authenticity. Through the compelling narrative of Sarah, readers are invited to embark on a poignant exploration of the complexities of weight management, emotional well-being, and the pursuit of a life that honors the intricacies of the human experience. Join us as we delve into Sarah's story, a testament to the transformative power of resilience and the profound impact of self-awareness on the path to personal growth and fulfillment.

Chapter 1:

STRUGGLES WITH WEIGHT

Sarah Davis sat on the edge of her bed, the morning sunlight filtering through the curtains, casting a soft glow over the cluttered room. Her tired eyes swept across the floor, skimming over discarded clothing and empty food wrappers scattered haphazardly. In the mirror opposite her, she caught a glimpse of her reflection. A sigh escaped her lips as she stared at the image that had become all too familiar - a figure she no longer recognized, cloaked in layers of excess weight.As the warmth of the morning sun slowly enveloped her, Sarah's mind drifted back to the early days of her struggle. Flashbacks of childhood taunts and cruel remarks echoed in her ears, each word a relentless reminder of the uphill battle she had faced. The playground jeers, the whispers in the school hallways - they had all left an indelible mark on her psyche. Sarah had grown up feeling like an outsider, someone perpetually on the fringes of acceptance.Her journey into adolescence had only compounded the issue. Endless nights spent seeking solace in the confines of her room, the flickering glow of the television casting a comforting haze over her world. Food became her companion, her solace in moments of despair, and her refuge in times of loneliness. The taste of sugary treats and salty snacks became a balm for her wounded spirit, momentarily soothing the ache of rejection and isolation.Over the years, the numbers on the scale had steadily climbed, inching upwards with each passing day. Sarah's reflection in the mirror had become a constant source of disappointment and self-loathing, a reminder of her perceived failure. The extra pounds had become more than just physical weight; they had evolved into an emotional burden that she carried with her every waking moment.With a deep breath, Sarah rose from the bed, the determination in her eyes a glimmer of hope amidst the sea of despair. Today was the day she decided to take charge of her life, to reclaim her sense of self-worth, and to break free from the chains of her own making. She knew the path ahead would be arduous, filled with obstacles and self-doubt, but she was ready to confront the challenge head-on.As she made her way to the kitchen, her footsteps purposeful and resolute, Sarah resolved to embark on a journey of self-discovery and transformation. With the first rays of morning light filtering through the window, she began to envision a future where the weight of her past would no longer define her. It was time to rewrite her story, one step at a time, and reclaim the life she had always deserved.

Chapter 2:

THE DECISION TO MAKE A CHANGE

The sun had begun its slow descent, casting a warm, golden glow across the room as Sarah sat at her cluttered desk, surrounded by stacks of books and articles on nutrition and exercise. Her laptop screen flickered with an array of websites, each offering a different perspective on the journey she was about to embark upon. The room was filled with the scent of determination, the air heavy with the weight of her impending decision.Sarah's fingers danced across the keyboard, her mind racing with conflicting thoughts and emotions. The allure of familiar comforts beckoned to her, whispering seductively of the temporary reprieve that a bag of chips or a pint of ice cream could offer. But amidst the cacophony of cravings, a resolute voice within her rose above the chaos, urging her to take control of her destiny. With a deep breath, Sarah closed her eyes, her mind drifting back to the countless moments of despair and self-doubt that had plagued her for years. The memories of missed opportunities, of fleeting glances that spoke of pity rather than admiration, flooded her consciousness. She had grown tired of being held captive by her own insecurities, tired of being shackled to a body that no longer felt like her own. As she opened her eyes, her gaze fell upon a photograph tucked away amidst the clutter on her desk. It was a picture of a younger, happier version of herself - a time when the burdens of self-doubt had not yet weighed her down. The sight of her radiant smile, unmarred by the shadows of insecurity, served as a beacon of hope, a reminder of the person she once was and the person she aspired to become once more. In that moment, a surge of determination coursed through her veins, infusing her with a newfound sense of purpose. With trembling hands, she reached for a pen and a blank sheet of paper, and began to outline a plan - a roadmap to a better, healthier future. She jotted down her goals, both short-term and long-term, envisioning a life free from the constraints of her past.As the evening shadows deepened, Sarah's resolve only strengthened, fortified by the flickering flame of her newfound determination. She knew the road ahead would be fraught with challenges and temptations, but she was prepared to confront them head-on. With each stroke of the pen, she solidified her commitment to a lifestyle of balance and self-care, vowing to treat her body with the respect and kindness it deserved.With the final stroke of the pen, Sarah leaned back in her chair, a sense of liberation washing over her. The decision to make a change had been made, and she was ready to embrace the journey that lay ahead, one step at a time. With the weight of indecision lifted from her shoulders, she allowed herself to bask in the warmth of newfound hope, the promise of a brighter future illuminating her path.

Chapter 3:

UNDERSTANDING THE IMPORTANCE OF A BALANCED DIET

The soft morning light seeped through the curtains, casting a gentle glow over Sarah's kitchen as she stood amidst a sea of colorful fruits and vegetables, her gaze shifting from one food item to the next. The air was infused with the tantalizing aroma of fresh produce, a welcome departure from the processed and packaged snacks that had dominated her pantry for far too long.As she surveyed the vibrant array before her, Sarah's mind began to unravel the complexities of what constituted a balanced diet. Memories of crash diets and extreme measures that had promised miraculous results flooded her thoughts, each one a stark reminder of the unsustainable practices she had once clung to in a desperate bid to shed unwanted pounds.With a renewed sense of purpose, Sarah set out to educate herself, diving headfirst into a world of nutritional knowledge and dietary wisdom. She devoured books and online resources, immersing herself in the intricacies of macronutrients and micronutrients, seeking to understand the fundamental building blocks that would fuel her journey towards a healthier lifestyle.As she pored over the pages, a newfound appreciation for the delicate balance of proteins, carbohydrates, and fats began to take root within her. She learned that each nutrient played a crucial role in supporting the body's functions, from energy production to immune system regulation. The revelation that food was not merely a source of momentary pleasure, but rather a cornerstone of vitality and well-being, ignited a spark of enthusiasm within her.Sarah's kitchen soon became a laboratory of experimentation, as she experimented with new recipes and culinary techniques, blending flavors and textures in a harmonious symphony of nourishment. She discovered the joys of incorporating a diverse array of whole foods into her meals, relishing the crisp crunch of leafy greens, the velvety richness of avocados, and the burst of sweetness from ripe berries.With each carefully curated meal, Sarah began to witness the transformative power of a balanced diet unfold before her eyes. Her energy levels surged, her mood stabilized, and her once-fickle digestion found equilibrium. The persistent cravings that had once held her captive began to wane, replaced by a newfound sense of satiety and satisfaction that transcended the fleeting allure of sugary indulgences.As she savored the flavors of her newly crafted meals, Sarah marveled at the intricate interplay of nutrients that had become the cornerstone of her rejuvenated lifestyle. She realized that a balanced diet was not merely a collection of food groups, but rather a holistic approach to nourishing both the body and the soul. With each bite, she felt a profound sense of gratitude for the transformative journey she had embarked upon, a journey that had unveiled the profound significance of mindful and deliberate nutrition.

Chapter 4:

SETTING REALISTIC GOALS AND PLANNING FOR SUCCESS

The faint scent of freshly brewed coffee lingered in the air as Sarah sat at her kitchen table, a notebook open before her, its blank pages waiting to be filled with the promises of a brighter future. She sipped her coffee slowly, savoring the rich warmth that spread through her body, igniting a sense of clarity and purpose within her.With determined eyes, she began to outline her aspirations, carefully delineating the steps that would pave the way for her journey towards a healthier and happier self. She understood the importance of setting realistic goals, of crafting a roadmap that would guide her through the inevitable peaks and valleys of her transformation.As she jotted down her initial thoughts, Sarah's mind raced with visions of

what she hoped to achieve. She envisioned a
future where each milestone conquered would
serve as a testament to her unwavering
commitment and resilience. She knew that the
path ahead would be riddled with challenges, but
she was determined not to let the fear of failure
deter her from her ultimate objective.With a
deep breath, she began to break down her
overarching goals into smaller, more
manageable targets. She understood the
significance of incremental progress, of
celebrating each small victory as a testament to
her unwavering dedication. Sarah knew that the
key to long-term success lay in the cultivation of
sustainable habits, in fostering a lifestyle that
would endure beyond the confines of a fleeting
moment of triumph.As she crafted her plan,
Sarah found herself gravitating towards the
concept of SMART goals - specific, measurable,
achievable, relevant, and time-bound. Each goal
she set was imbued with a sense of purpose and
direction, each milestone etched with the clarity
of intention and the determination to
succeed.With each goal outlined, Sarah's sense

of empowerment grew, bolstered by the knowledge that she held the reins to her own destiny. She understood that her journey was not merely about shedding pounds, but rather about cultivating a mindset of self-compassion and resilience, one that would carry her through the inevitable setbacks and obstacles that lay ahead.As she put the finishing touches on her plan, Sarah felt a surge of confidence course through her veins, a sense of conviction that she was on the right path towards a brighter and healthier future. With her goals set and her roadmap in hand, she leaned back in her chair, a smile of quiet determination gracing her lips. She was ready to embrace the challenges that lay ahead, armed with a clear vision of the success that awaited her at the end of her transformative journey.

Chapter 5:

OVERCOMING TEMPTATION AND EMOTIONAL EATING

The evening sun cast long shadows across Sarah's kitchen, the faint aroma of freshly baked cookies lingering in the air. She stood by the counter, her fingers hovering over the plate of warm treats, her resolve wavering in the face of familiar temptation. Her mind was a whirlwind of conflicting emotions, the allure of a momentary indulgence threatening to unravel the progress she had painstakingly built.As she hesitated, Sarah's thoughts drifted back to the countless times she had sought solace in the embrace of comfort food, the sugary sweetness and the familiar crunch a temporary respite from the chaos of her emotions. She recalled the moments of despair and loneliness that had driven her to seek refuge in the confines of her pantry, the rhythmic motion of her hand to mouth providing a fleeting distraction from the ache of her heart.With a heavy sigh, Sarah reached for a notepad and pen, determined to confront the source of her emotional eating. She began to jot down the triggers that had consistently lured her into the familiar cycle of consumption - moments of stress, feelings of inadequacy, and the relentless pursuit of fleeting pleasure. She understood that her relationship with food transcended mere sustenance; it had become a complex tapestry of emotional entanglement that required careful unraveling.As she traced the patterns of her behavior, Sarah began to unearth the underlying emotions that had driven her to seek refuge in the arms of food. She acknowledged the pain of past traumas that had yet to heal, the insecurities that had taken root in the fertile soil of her self-doubt. With each stroke of the pen, she peeled back the layers of her psyche, exposing the vulnerabilities that had long been shielded from the light of day.Armed with a newfound sense of self-awareness, Sarah resolved to develop coping mechanisms that did not rely on the temporary relief of emotional eating. She turned to the soothing embrace of mindfulness and meditation, embracing the healing power of self-reflection and introspection. She sought solace in the company of loved ones, fostering connections that nourished her spirit and provided a sense of belonging and acceptance.As she embarked on this journey of self-discovery, Sarah learned to recognize the warning signs of impending emotional eating, to identify the moments when her cravings were merely a manifestation of unresolved turmoil. She armed herself with a repertoire of healthier alternatives, from engaging in physical activity to immersing herself in creative pursuits, each one serving as a beacon of light amidst the shadows of her emotional landscape.With each passing day, Sarah felt the tendrils of temptation loosen their grip on her, their once-pervasive influence waning in the face of her unwavering determination. She understood that the road to overcoming emotional eating would be paved with moments of vulnerability and uncertainty, but she was resolute in her commitment to reclaim control over her relationship with food. As she set the plate of untouched cookies aside, a sense of triumph washed over her, a testament to the strength and resilience that lay dormant within her. She was ready to confront the challenges that lay ahead, armed with the knowledge that she held the power to rewrite her narrative and forge a healthier, more empowered future.

Chapter 6:

DISCOVERING THE POWER OF
PORTION CONTROL

The midday sun filtered through the curtains, casting a warm glow over Sarah's dining table, which was adorned with an array of colorful dishes. Her gaze swept over the spread before her, each plate brimming with a carefully measured serving of food. As she reached for her fork, she marveled at the newfound sense of empowerment that came with the practice of portion control, a concept that had once eluded her in the haze of mindless consumption.With each bite, Sarah savored the flavors dancing on her palate, the careful balance of textures and spices a testament to the art of mindful eating. She had come to understand that portion control was not about deprivation, but rather about fostering a harmonious relationship with food, one that honored both the body's nutritional needs and the soul's desire for nourishment.As she reflected on her journey, Sarah traced back to the pivotal moment when she had first recognized the significance of portion control. She recalled the years of overindulgence and unchecked consumption, the absence of restraint and the resulting weight gain that had left her feeling imprisoned within her own body. It was a journey fraught with excess, a path that had led her to confront the harsh reality of her unsustainable habits.With a determined spirit, Sarah had delved into the intricacies of portion control, immersing herself in the knowledge of serving sizes and nutritional guidelines. She learned to decipher the subtle cues that signaled satiety, to discern the delicate balance between nourishment and overconsumption. With each meal, she honed her ability to gauge her body's needs, to listen to the whispers of hunger and fullness that had long been drowned out by the clamor of her cravings.As she integrated portion control into her daily routine, Sarah witnessed a gradual transformation take root within her. She began to feel a newfound sense of lightness, both physical and emotional, as the burden of overeating was replaced by the liberation of mindful moderation. She discovered that a smaller, well-portioned meal could satiate her just as effectively as a larger, unchecked feast, and that the key to satisfaction lay not in the quantity of food, but in the quality of the experience.With each passing day, Sarah's mastery of portion control became second nature, a seamless integration of a practice that had once seemed daunting and unfamiliar. She understood that her journey was not merely about the number on the scale, but rather about fostering a sense of balance and harmony that extended far beyond the confines of her plate. As she savored the final morsels of her carefully curated meal, a sense of gratitude washed over her, a testament to the transformative power of mindful consumption and the profound impact it had on her journey towards a healthier and more fulfilling life.

Chapter 7:

EXPLORING DIFFERENT DIETING TECHNIQUES

Sarah sat at her desk, surrounded by a stack of books and research papers, her brow furrowed in deep concentration as she delved into the diverse landscape of dieting techniques. Her quest for a sustainable and effective approach to weight management had led her to explore the myriad strategies and philosophies that promised a path to a healthier lifestyle. With an open mind and a discerning eye, she began to navigate the intricate maze of dieting methodologies, seeking to unearth the practices that would resonate most deeply with her journey.As she combed through the wealth of information before her, Sarah encountered a kaleidoscope of dieting techniques, each one bearing its own unique set of principles and promises. She learned about the merits of the ketogenic diet, which emphasized the consumption of healthy fats and minimal carbohydrates, plunging the body into a state of ketosis that facilitated fat burning and weight loss. She discovered the virtues of the Mediterranean diet, with its emphasis on whole grains, fruits, vegetables, and lean proteins, rooted in the culinary traditions of the Mediterranean region and heralded for its heart-healthy benefits.Sarah delved into the intricacies of intermittent fasting, an approach that entailed cycling between periods of eating and fasting, with the potential to regulate blood sugar levels and promote cellular repair and regeneration. She explored the principles of the paleo diet, which advocated for a return to the dietary habits of our ancient ancestors, emphasizing the consumption of whole, unprocessed foods and the exclusion of grains, legumes, and dairy products.As she absorbed the nuances of each dieting technique, Sarah began to discern the common threads that wove through the fabric of these disparate methodologies. She recognized the importance of prioritizing whole, nutrient-dense foods, of cultivating a diet rich in fruits, vegetables, and lean proteins that nourished the body from within. She understood that the key to sustainable weight management lay not in adhering to a rigid set of rules, but rather in fostering a flexible and intuitive approach that honored the body's unique needs and preferences.Armed with a comprehensive understanding of the diverse dieting techniques at her disposal, Sarah began to weave together a tapestry of practices that resonated most deeply with her journey. She embraced the principles of balance and moderation, integrating elements from various methodologies to craft a personalized approach that spoke to her individuality and her aspirations for a healthier and more vibrant life.As she closed the final book and set aside the last research paper, Sarah felt a profound sense of empowerment wash over her, a testament to the knowledge and wisdom she had gained throughout her exploration. She understood that her journey was not bound by the confines of a single doctrine, but rather shaped by the amalgamation of practices and principles that had resonated most deeply with her quest for holistic well-being. With newfound clarity and purpose, she set out to implement her learnings, embracing a comprehensive approach to dieting that honored the intricate interplay of nourishment, vitality, and self-discovery.

Chapter 8:

INCORPORATING EXERCISE INTO DAILY LIFE

The first rays of dawn peeked over the horizon as Sarah laced up her running shoes, her breath forming delicate puffs of mist in the crisp morning air. With each stride, she felt the rhythm of her heartbeat synchronize with the cadence of her footsteps, the steady tempo of her breath a testament to the power of movement and vitality. She had come to understand that exercise was not merely a chore to be checked off a list, but rather a transformative practice that infused her days with energy and purpose.As Sarah embarked on her daily run, she reminisced about the initial trepidation she had felt at the prospect of incorporating exercise into her routine. She recalled the echoes of doubt and self-consciousness that had once lingered at the periphery of her consciousness, the fear of judgment and the discomfort of unfamiliarity threatening to impede her progress. But with each passing day, she had learned to embrace the discomfort, to lean into the challenges that lay before her, and to discover the joy and liberation that came with pushing her boundaries and surpassing her limitations.Through trial and error, Sarah had explored a myriad of exercise modalities, from high-intensity interval training to yoga, from weightlifting to swimming. She had discovered the unique joys and benefits that each form of exercise offered, from the adrenaline rush of a heart-pounding workout to the serene tranquility of a meditative yoga practice. She understood that exercise was not confined to the boundaries of a gym; it was a versatile and dynamic practice that could be woven seamlessly into the fabric of her daily life.With each passing week, Sarah felt her body grow stronger, more resilient, and more attuned to the demands of physical exertion. She marveled at the newfound agility and flexibility that had blossomed within her, the once-familiar limitations of her body giving way to the boundless potential that lay dormant within her. She understood that exercise was not merely a means to an end, but rather a holistic practice that nurtured her physical, mental, and emotional well-being, fostering a sense of balance and harmony that transcended the confines of her physical form.As she completed her morning run and made her way back home, Sarah felt a surge of exhilaration wash over her, a sense of accomplishment that reverberated through every fiber of her being. She understood that exercise had become more than just a habit; it had evolved into a lifeline that buoyed her spirit and fueled her passion for life. With each passing day, she looked forward to the moments of movement and exertion that awaited her, knowing that each step, each stretch, and each breath brought her closer to a sense of vitality and fulfillment that transcended the boundaries of her wildest dreams.

Chapter 9:

MANAGING STRESS AND ITS IMPACT ON WEIGHT LOSS

The gentle hum of a meditation app filled the air as Sarah sat cross-legged on her yoga mat, her eyes closed, her mind enveloped in a cocoon of tranquility. With each inhale and exhale, she felt the weight of the world begin to lift from her shoulders, the knots of tension that had once bound her spirit slowly unraveling in the embrace of mindfulness and stillness. She had come to understand that stress was not merely an emotional burden, but rather a physical and psychological disruptor that could impede her journey towards holistic well-being.As she delved into the intricacies of stress management, Sarah began to recognize the profound impact that stress could have on her body and, by extension, her weight loss journey. She learned that chronic stress could trigger the release of cortisol, a hormone that, when produced in excess, could lead to an increase in appetite and the accumulation of abdominal fat. She discovered that the relentless demands of modern life had left her perpetually teetering on the edge of a precipice, her equilibrium threatened by the ceaseless onslaught of external pressures and internal turmoil.With a newfound sense of urgency, Sarah immersed herself in the practice of stress-reduction techniques, seeking solace in the healing embrace of meditation, yoga, and deep breathing exercises. She explored the restorative powers of nature, allowing the soothing whispers of the wind and the gentle rustle of leaves to lull her into a state of serenity and calm. She embraced the therapeutic benefits of journaling, allowing the ink to flow freely as she unburdened her thoughts and emotions onto the pages before her.As she integrated these practices into her daily routine, Sarah began to witness a gradual transformation take root within her. She felt the tendrils of stress loosen their grip on her, their once-omnipresent influence waning in the face of her newfound resilience and inner peace. She learned to confront the sources of her stress with a sense of equanimity and detachment, understanding that her reactions to external stimuli were within her control, even when the circumstances themselves were not. With each passing day, Sarah felt a renewed sense of vitality and clarity take hold of her, a sense of empowerment that stemmed from her ability to navigate the turbulent waters of stress with grace and fortitude. She understood that the journey towards weight loss was not merely a physical endeavor, but rather a holistic transformation that encompassed the nurturing of her mind, body, and spirit. As she rose from her meditation, a serene smile graced her lips, a testament to the profound impact that stress management had had on her journey towards a healthier and more balanced life.

Chapter 10:

DEALING WITH PLATEAUS AND STAYING MOTIVATED

The dim light of dawn filtered through the window, casting long shadows across the room as Sarah stood on the scale, her heart sinking at the sight of the unchanging number before her. She had hit a plateau, a stagnant stretch in her weight loss journey that seemed to mock her efforts and test her resilience. Her mind swirled with doubt and frustration, the once-familiar sense of progress and accomplishment now replaced by a cloud of uncertainty and stagnation.As she grappled with the reality of her plateau, Sarah's thoughts drifted back to the moments of triumph that had punctuated her journey. She recalled the initial surge of motivation that had propelled her forward, the sense of purpose and determination that had fueled her every step and every choice. But now, faced with the stubborn resistance of her body, she found herself at a crossroads, grappling with the harsh truth that progress was not always linear, and that setbacks were an inevitable part of the transformative process.With a deep breath, Sarah resolved to confront her plateau with unwavering determination and resilience. She understood that the key to overcoming this obstacle lay not in succumbing to despair, but rather in embracing a multifaceted approach that addressed both the physical and psychological dimensions of her journey. She delved into the nuances of her diet and exercise regimen, seeking to identify potential areas for adjustment and refinement that could reignite the flames of progress within her.As she grappled with the challenges of her plateau, Sarah sought solace in the company of her support system, leaning on the unwavering encouragement and guidance of her loved ones. She found inspiration in the stories of others who had faced similar obstacles and emerged triumphant, their tales serving as a beacon of hope and resilience amidst the shadows of her uncertainty. She understood that the journey towards sustainable weight loss was not without its pitfalls and roadblocks, but that each setback was an opportunity for growth and self-discovery, a chance to cultivate a deeper sense of fortitude and perseverance. With each passing day, Sarah rekindled the flames of her motivation, stoking the embers of her determination and commitment with the knowledge that her plateau was not a reflection of her inadequacy, but rather a testament to the intricacies of the human body and its propensity for adaptation. She understood that the road ahead would be paved with moments of uncertainty and doubt, but that her unwavering resolve would guide her through the darkest valleys and lead her to the triumphant peaks that awaited her on the other side. As she stepped off the scale, a sense of renewed determination coursed through her veins, a silent vow to confront her plateau with grace and resilience, and to emerge stronger and more resilient than ever before.

Chapter 11:

EXPLORING THE BENEFITS OF MEAL PREPPING

Sarah stood in her kitchen, a whirlwind of activity swirling around her as she meticulously measured and chopped an array of fresh produce. The scent of herbs and spices infused the air, creating a symphony of flavors that hinted at the culinary delights to come. With each deft movement of her knife, she marveled at the transformative power of meal prepping, a practice that had revolutionized her approach to nutrition and time management.As she crafted each dish with care and precision, Sarah began to unravel the myriad benefits of meal prepping that had become the cornerstone of her culinary journey. She discovered that meal prepping not only saved her time and energy throughout the week, but also empowered her to make mindful and nourishing choices that supported her weight loss goals. She realized that the practice of planning and preparing her meals in advance instilled a sense of discipline and structure that permeated every facet of her daily life.With a pantry stocked with carefully curated ingredients and a menu meticulously planned for the week ahead, Sarah found herself liberated from the clutches of impulsive and haphazard eating. She reveled in the convenience of having nutritious meals readily available, each one a testament to her commitment to fostering a lifestyle of balance and well-being. She understood that meal prepping was not merely about convenience, but rather a holistic practice that nurtured her body and nourished her soul, one carefully portioned container at a time.As she organized her neatly arranged meals in the refrigerator, Sarah marveled at the versatility and creativity that meal prepping had unlocked within her. She experimented with an array of flavors and cuisines, infusing each dish with a sense of excitement and anticipation that transcended the mundane act of consumption.

She found joy in the rhythmic dance of preparation, in the symphony of colors and textures that adorned her plate, and in the knowledge that each meal was a celebration of her commitment to self-care and holistic well-being.With each passing day, Sarah witnessed the transformative power of meal prepping unfold before her eyes, a testament to the profound impact that mindful and deliberate nutrition could have on her journey towards a healthier and more vibrant life. She understood that meal prepping was not merely a chore, but rather a ritual of self-love and nourishment, a practice that honored the intricate interplay of nourishment, vitality, and culinary artistry. As she surveyed the neatly arranged containers before her, a sense of satisfaction washed over her, a quiet affirmation of the profound benefits that meal prepping had brought to her life and her journey towards sustainable weight loss and holistic well-being.

Chapter 12:

THE ROLE OF SLEEP IN WEIGHT MANAGEMENT

The moon hung low in the night sky as Sarah settled into her bed, the soft embrace of her pillows and blankets cocooning her in a sanctuary of tranquility. With each slow, deep breath, she felt the tendrils of sleep envelop her, gently carrying her away to a realm of serenity and rest. As she drifted into the embrace of slumber, she marveled at the profound impact that sleep had on her journey towards sustainable weight management.In the light of day, Sarah delved into the intricate nuances of the relationship between sleep and weight management, seeking to unravel the complex interplay of hormones and physiological processes that governed her body's response to rest and wakefulness. She learned that sleep played a pivotal role in regulating the hormones that controlled her appetite, with insufficient sleep leading to an increase in the production of ghrelin, the hormone that stimulated hunger, and a decrease in the production of leptin, the hormone that signaled satiety.As she delved deeper into her research, Sarah discovered that the effects of sleep deprivation extended beyond mere fluctuations in appetite. She learned that inadequate sleep disrupted the body's metabolic processes, leading to a decrease in insulin sensitivity and an increase in blood sugar levels, which could ultimately contribute to weight gain and the development of metabolic disorders. She understood that the repercussions of poor sleep extended far beyond the realms of physical health, manifesting in cognitive impairments, emotional instability, and a diminished capacity for self-regulation and decision-making.Armed with this knowledge, Sarah endeavored to prioritize her sleep hygiene, cultivating a bedtime routine that fostered a sense of relaxation and tranquility. She created a soothing environment in her bedroom, free from the disruptive glow of electronic screens and the clamor of external stimuli. She embraced the therapeutic benefits of meditation and deep breathing exercises, allowing the rhythmic cadence of her breath to lull her into a state of calm and equilibrium.With each night of restful slumber, Sarah felt the transformative power of sleep infuse her days with newfound energy and vitality. She witnessed the subtle shifts in her appetite and her cravings, the sense of balance and satiety that accompanied her meals, and the clarity of mind and emotional resilience that permeated her interactions and decision-making processes. She understood that sleep was not merely a luxury, but rather a cornerstone of holistic well-being, a practice that nurtured her body, mind, and spirit and laid the foundation for sustainable weight management and a vibrant, fulfilling life. As she embraced the transformative power of rest, Sarah marveled at the profound impact that sleep had on her journey towards holistic health and wellness, understanding that each night of peaceful slumber was a silent affirmation of the body's

innate wisdom and its capacity for rejuvenation
and renewal.

Chapter 13:

NAVIGATING SOCIAL SITUATIONS AND EATING OUT

Sarah stood amidst a bustling restaurant, the tantalizing aroma of freshly prepared dishes wafting through the air, the rhythmic hum of conversation enveloping her in a warm embrace. As she perused the menu before her, her mind raced with conflicting thoughts and emotions, grappling with the familiar challenge of making mindful and nourishing choices in the midst of a social setting. She had come to understand that navigating social situations and eating out was not merely about adhering to a set of dietary restrictions, but rather about fostering a sense of balance and moderation that honored both her health goals and her need for human connection and camaraderie. With a deep breath, Sarah resolved to approach the dining experience with a sense of mindfulness and intention. She perused the menu with a discerning eye, seeking out dishes that balanced nutritional value with sensory delight, each one a testament to her commitment to nourishing her body and soul. She engaged in open and honest communication with her companions, sharing her dietary preferences and goals with grace and confidence, and inviting them to join her on a journey towards healthier and more conscious eating.As she engaged in conversation and laughter with her companions, Sarah learned to savor each bite, to relish the flavors and textures that graced her palate, and to cultivate a sense of gratitude for the culinary delights that enriched her social experiences. She understood that eating out was not merely a transactional act of consumption, but rather a communal celebration of culture, tradition, and shared experiences, each meal a reflection of the diverse tapestry of human connection and camaraderie.Armed with a sense of empowerment and self-assurance, Sarah found joy in the art of adaptation, learning to navigate the intricate terrain of social situations and eating out with grace and resilience. She discovered the myriad ways in which she could make informed and nourishing choices without sacrificing the pleasures of indulgence and exploration, balancing moments of restraint with moments of celebration and delight. She understood that the journey towards sustainable weight management was not about isolating herself from the world, but rather about fostering a harmonious relationship with food that honored both her individuality and her interconnectedness with the world around her.With each shared meal and each heartfelt conversation, Sarah felt the bonds of community and camaraderie grow stronger, her journey towards holistic well-being enriched by the connections she forged and the memories she created. She understood that the path to sustainable weight management was not a solitary one, but rather a collective endeavor that thrived on the bonds of understanding, support, and shared aspirations. As she bid her companions farewell and stepped out into the bustling streets, a sense of contentment washed over her, a quiet affirmation of the transformative power of mindful and conscious eating in the tapestry of human connection and the joys of communal celebration.

Chapter 14:

UNDERSTANDING NUTRITIONAL LABELS AND MAKING INFORMED CHOICES

Sarah stood in the aisle of her local grocery store, a meticulously designed package clutched in her hand, her eyes scanning the intricate web of numbers and figures that adorned the label before her. With a furrowed brow, she delved into the nuances of the nutritional information, seeking to unravel the hidden truths and revelations that lay beneath the surface. She had come to understand that the practice of deciphering nutritional labels was not merely a matter of perfunctory glances, but rather a skill that empowered her to make informed and nourishing choices that aligned with her health goals and aspirations.As she immersed herself in the complexities of the label, Sarah learned to discern the key components that dictated the nutritional value of the product. She identified the significance of serving sizes, understanding that the values listed on the label were often contingent on specific portion sizes that could vary from one product to another. She delved into the intricacies of macronutrients - carbohydrates, fats, and proteins - recognizing their distinct roles in fueling the body's functions and understanding the implications of their consumption on her overall health and well-being.Armed with a comprehensive understanding of the nutritional label, Sarah began to navigate the aisles of the grocery store with a discerning eye, selecting products that aligned with her dietary preferences and nutritional requirements. She learned to identify hidden sugars and artificial additives, recognizing their potential impact on her energy levels and overall health. She sought out products that boasted a rich array of vitamins, minerals, and antioxidants, understanding that the key to optimal nutrition lay not in the absence of certain ingredients, but rather in the abundance of wholesome and nourishing components that supported her journey towards holistic well-being. With each product carefully scrutinized and each label meticulously analyzed, Sarah felt a sense of empowerment and autonomy blossom within her. She understood that the practice of deciphering nutritional labels was not merely a means to an end, but rather a cornerstone of informed decision-making and self-care. She recognized that her ability to make conscious and deliberate choices at the grocery store transcended the realms of dieting and weight management, permeating every facet of her lifestyle and underscoring her commitment to nurturing a body, mind, and spirit that thrived on the abundance of wholesome and nourishing nourishment. As she filled her shopping cart with a bountiful array of nutrient-dense products, Sarah felt a profound sense of gratitude wash over her, a quiet affirmation of the transformative power of understanding nutritional labels and making informed choices.

She understood that each selection she made was not merely a transactional act of consumption, but rather a declaration of her unwavering commitment to self-awareness, self-empowerment, and the pursuit of holistic well-being.

Chapter 15:

EMBRACING A SUSTAINABLE AND LONG-TERM APPROACH

Sarah sat at her desk, her gaze fixed on the blank page before her, her mind a whirlwind of thoughts and reflections as she contemplated the profound impact of her weight management journey. With each keystroke, she sought to capture the essence of her transformation, to distill the wisdom and insights that had guided her towards a path of sustainable and long-term wellness. She had come to understand that the pursuit of weight management was not merely a fleeting endeavor, but rather a lifelong commitment to nurturing a lifestyle that honored the intricate interplay of nourishment, vitality, and self-discovery.As she delved into the intricacies of sustainable weight management, Sarah learned to cultivate a holistic approach that encompassed the dimensions of physical, mental, and emotional well-being. She understood that the key to sustainable success lay not in the adoption of rigid and restrictive practices, but rather in the cultivation of a flexible and intuitive mindset that honored the body's innate wisdom and its capacity for balance and self-regulation.Armed with this knowledge, Sarah endeavored to integrate sustainable practices into every facet of her daily life, from the foods she consumed to the activities she engaged in, and the thoughts she cultivated. She learned to foster a sense of mindfulness and intention in her dietary choices, embracing a diverse array of nutrient-dense foods that nourished her body from within. She cultivated a regular exercise routine that brought joy and vitality into her days, understanding that movement was not merely a means to an end, but rather a celebration of the body's strength and resilience.As she grappled with the challenges and triumphs of her journey, Sarah found solace in the unwavering support of her community, leaning on the wisdom and encouragement of her loved ones to bolster her spirits and reaffirm her commitment to holistic well-being. She understood that the road to sustainable weight management was not without its setbacks and obstacles, but that each moment of adversity was an opportunity for growth and self-discovery, a chance to cultivate a deeper sense of resilience and fortitude.With each passing day, Sarah felt the transformative power of her sustainable approach infuse her life with a newfound sense of vitality and purpose. She marveled at the resilience and grace that had blossomed within her, the once-familiar shadows of doubt and uncertainty now replaced by the radiant light of self-empowerment and self-acceptance. She understood that her journey was not merely about shedding pounds, but rather about embracing a lifestyle that honored her body, mind, and spirit, and celebrated the boundless potential that resided within her. As she penned the final words of her narrative, a sense of tranquility washed over her, a silent affirmation of the transformative power of embracing a sustainable and long-term approach to weight management, and the profound impact it had on her journey towards holistic well-being and a life of purpose and vitality.

Chapter 16:

CONFRONTING BODY IMAGE ISSUES AND BUILDING SELF-CONFIDENCE

Sarah stood before the mirror, her gaze tracing the contours of her reflection, her mind a tumultuous sea of conflicting emotions and perceptions. With each passing moment, she grappled with the harsh realities of body image issues, the echoes of self-doubt and insecurity that had long plagued her sense of self-worth and belonging. But amidst the shadows of uncertainty, she had come to understand that the journey towards building self-confidence was not merely about physical transformation, but rather a profound exploration of self-acceptance, resilience, and inner strength.As she embarked on her journey of self-discovery, Sarah delved into the depths of her psyche, seeking to unravel the origins of her body image issues and the societal constructs that had shaped her perceptions of beauty and worth. She confronted the lingering echoes of comparison and self-criticism, understanding that her value as an individual was not contingent on external standards of perfection, but rather on the unique tapestry of experiences, aspirations, and resilience that defined her essence.Armed with a newfound sense of self-awareness and compassion, Sarah cultivated a practice of self-love and acceptance that extended beyond the confines of her physical form. She learned to celebrate her body as a vessel of resilience and vitality, a testament to the countless moments of triumph and perseverance that had shaped her journey towards holistic well-being. She understood that her imperfections were not flaws to be hidden or erased, but rather a testament to the beauty of human authenticity and the capacity for growth and self-empowerment.With each passing day, Sarah embraced a narrative of self-confidence and empowerment, challenging the confines of societal norms and expectations with a spirit of defiance and resilience. She surrounded herself with a community of individuals who celebrated diversity and individuality, fostering a sense of belonging and acceptance that transcended the limitations of external judgment and scrutiny. She recognized that the journey towards building self-confidence was not a solitary one, but rather a collective endeavor that thrived on the bonds of empathy, understanding, and shared aspirations.As she stood before the mirror once more, Sarah felt a surge of gratitude wash over her, a quiet affirmation of the transformative power of self-acceptance and self-confidence. She understood that her journey was not merely about confronting body image issues, but rather about embracing a narrative of self-love and empowerment that honored her individuality and celebrated the boundless potential that resided within her. With a renewed sense of purpose and vitality, she stepped away from the mirror, a radiant smile gracing her lips, a testament to the profound impact that confronting body image issues and building self-confidence had on her journey towards holistic well-being and a life of purpose and authenticity.

Chapter 17:

THE IMPACT OF SUPPORT SYSTEMS AND COMMUNITY ON WEIGHT LOSS

Sarah sat amidst a circle of kindred spirits, the warmth of their camaraderie and understanding enveloping her in a comforting embrace. With each shared story and each heartfelt exchange, she marveled at the transformative power of support systems and community on her journey towards sustainable weight loss. She had come to understand that the bonds of empathy and understanding were not merely superficial connections, but rather lifelines that buoyed her spirit and fueled her passion for self-discovery and holistic well-being.As she delved into the intricacies of her support system, Sarah recognized the profound impact that the unwavering encouragement and guidance of her loved ones had on her journey. She understood that the shared experiences and collective wisdom of her community offered a sanctuary of understanding and solace, a space where she could freely express her triumphs and tribulations without fear of judgment or reproach. She found strength in the stories of others who had faced similar challenges and emerged triumphant, their tales serving as a beacon of hope and resilience amidst the shadows of her uncertainty.Armed with the nurturing embrace of her support system, Sarah felt a profound sense of empowerment and camaraderie blossom within her. She learned to lean on the wisdom and guidance of her loved ones, seeking solace in their unwavering encouragement and belief in her journey. She found inspiration in their shared aspirations and triumphs, understanding that the road to sustainable weight loss was not a solitary one, but rather a collective endeavor that thrived on the bonds of empathy, understanding, and shared aspirations.With each passing day, Sarah felt the transformative power of her community infuse her life with a newfound sense of vitality and purpose. She marveled at the resilience and grace that had blossomed within her, the once-familiar shadows of doubt and uncertainty now replaced by the radiant light of camaraderie and shared triumph. She understood that her journey was not merely about shedding pounds, but rather about embracing a narrative of resilience and communal support that honored her individuality and celebrated the boundless potential that resided within her.As she bid her companions farewell and stepped out into the world, a sense of contentment washed over her, a quiet affirmation of the transformative power of support systems and community on her journey towards holistic well-being and a life of purpose and vitality. She understood that each connection she forged was not merely a transactional bond, but rather a lifeline that buoyed her spirit and fueled her passion for self-discovery and the pursuit of a life that thrived on the nurturing embrace of community and shared resilience.

Chapter 18:

COPING WITH SETBACKS AND REGAINING FOCUS

Sarah sat at her desk, the weight of disappointment and frustration settling heavily upon her shoulders, her mind a whirlwind of doubts and uncertainties. With each passing moment, she grappled with the harsh reality of setbacks, the familiar shadows of self-doubt and discouragement threatening to derail her journey towards sustainable weight management. But amidst the darkness, she had come to understand that the key to resilience lay not in the absence of adversity, but rather in the tenacity and determination with which she confronted and navigated the challenges that lay before her.As she delved into the intricacies of coping with setbacks, Sarah cultivated a practice of self-compassion and understanding that extended beyond the realms of external validation and achievement. She learned to embrace the lessons embedded within moments of adversity, recognizing that each setback was an opportunity for growth and self-discovery, a chance to cultivate a deeper sense of resilience and self-awareness. She understood that the journey towards sustainable weight management was not without its trials and tribulations, but that each moment of uncertainty was an invitation to reclaim her sense of purpose and rekindle the flames of her determination.Armed with this knowledge, Sarah endeavored to reframe her perception of setbacks, understanding that they were not indicators of inadequacy or failure, but rather stepping stones towards a deeper understanding of her strengths and capabilities. She sought solace in the unwavering support of her community, leaning on the wisdom and encouragement of her loved ones to bolster her spirits and reaffirm her commitment to self-care and holistic well-being. She understood that the road to resilience was not a solitary one, but rather a collective endeavor that thrived on the bonds of empathy, understanding, and shared aspirations.With each passing day, Sarah felt the transformative power of her resilience infuse her life with a newfound sense of vitality and purpose. She marveled at the strength and grace that had blossomed within her, the once-familiar shadows of doubt and uncertainty now replaced by the radiant light of self-empowerment and self-acceptance. She understood that her journey was not merely about confronting setbacks, but rather about embracing a narrative of perseverance and inner strength that honored her individuality and celebrated the boundless potential that resided within her.As she turned her gaze towards the future, a sense of tranquility washed over her, a silent affirmation of the transformative power of coping with setbacks and regaining focus. She understood that each moment of uncertainty was not a roadblock, but rather a catalyst for growth and self-discovery, a chance to cultivate a deeper sense of resilience and self-awareness that would guide her through the darkest valleys and lead

her to the triumphant peaks that awaited her on
the other side.

Chapter 19:

EXPLORING DIFFERENT TYPES OF WORKOUTS AND EXERCISE ROUTINES

Sarah stood at the threshold of her gym, the air alive with the rhythmic cadence of movement and exertion, the faint echoes of laughter and determination enveloping her in a cocoon of vitality and purpose. With each step, she delved into the vibrant tapestry of exercise routines and workout regimens that awaited her, each one a unique exploration of the body's capacity for strength, flexibility, and endurance. She had come to understand that the path to holistic well-being was not limited to a singular form of exercise, but rather a diverse array of movements and activities that celebrated the intricacies of the human physique.As she immersed herself in the world of fitness, Sarah embraced a multifaceted approach that encompassed the realms of cardiovascular endurance, muscular strength, and flexibility. She delved into the nuances of aerobic exercises, reveling in the invigorating pulse of activities such as running, cycling, and swimming that bolstered her cardiovascular health and infused her days with a sense of vitality and resilience. She explored the realms of strength training, discovering the transformative power of weightlifting and resistance exercises that sculpted her physique and fortified her muscles with a newfound sense of power and resilience.Armed with a comprehensive understanding of the diverse array of exercise routines, Sarah delved into the realms of flexibility and mobility, embracing the therapeutic benefits of activities such as yoga, Pilates, and stretching that nurtured her body and soul with a sense of grace and equilibrium. She marveled at the profound impact that each form of exercise had on her physical and mental well-being, understanding that the key to holistic wellness lay not in the exclusivity of a singular routine, but rather in the integration of diverse movements and activities that honored the body's innate capacity for balance and vitality. With each workout and each exercise routine, Sarah felt the transformative power of movement infuse her life with a newfound sense of energy and purpose. She marveled at the resilience and grace that had blossomed within her, the once-familiar shadows of fatigue and lethargy now replaced by the radiant light of strength and vitality. She understood that her journey was not merely about adhering to a rigid and monotonous routine, but rather about embracing a narrative of diversity and exploration that celebrated the boundless potential of the human physique and the transformative power of movement. As she bid the gym farewell and stepped out into the world, a sense of contentment washed over her, a quiet affirmation of the profound impact that exploring different types of workouts and exercise routines had on her journey towards holistic well-being and a life of purpose and resilience.

Chapter 20:

RECOGNIZING AND AVOIDING FAD DIETS AND MISINFORMATION

Sarah sat at her desk, the glow of her laptop illuminating the contours of her determined expression as she delved into the intricate web of nutrition and dieting trends that populated the digital landscape before her. With each click and each scroll, she grappled with the pervasive presence of fad diets and misinformation that inundated her search results, the alluring promises of quick fixes and instant transformations tempting her with their mirage of effortless success. But amidst the cacophony of conflicting advice and sensationalist claims, she had come to understand that the pursuit of sustainable weight management was not a journey paved with shortcuts and magic bullets, but rather a nuanced exploration of self-awareness, resilience, and informed decision-making.As she delved into the depths of her research, Sarah learned to discern the telltale signs of fad diets, recognizing their propensity for extreme restrictions and unsustainable practices that often yielded short-term results at the cost of long-term well-being. She identified the sensationalist rhetoric and lofty promises that characterized their marketing strategies, understanding that their allure lay not in their efficacy, but rather in their ability to prey on the vulnerabilities and insecurities of individuals seeking a quick and effortless path to weight loss.Armed with this knowledge, Sarah cultivated a practice of critical thinking and discernment, learning to sift through the vast expanse of information and advice with a discerning eye and a sense of self-awareness. She sought out reputable sources and evidence-based research, understanding that the key to making informed and nourishing choices lay not in the embrace of fleeting trends, but rather in the integration of sustainable practices and holistic lifestyle modifications that honored the body's innate wisdom and its capacity for balance and well-being.With each passing day, Sarah felt the transformative power of her discernment infuse her life with a newfound sense of empowerment and resilience. She marveled at the strength and grace that had blossomed within her, the once-familiar shadows of confusion and uncertainty now replaced by the radiant light of self-awareness and informed decision-making. She understood that her journey was not merely about avoiding the pitfalls of fad diets and misinformation, but rather about embracing a narrative of self-empowerment and critical thinking that honored her individuality and celebrated the boundless potential that resided within her.As she closed her laptop and turned her gaze towards the future, a sense of tranquility washed over her, a silent affirmation of the transformative power of recognizing and avoiding fad diets and misinformation. She understood that each moment of discernment was not merely an act of skepticism, but rather a declaration of her unwavering commitment to self-awareness, resilience, and the pursuit of a life that thrived on the nourishing embrace of informed decision-making and holistic well-being.

Chapter 21:

CELEBRATING NON-SCALE VICTORIES AND PROGRESS

Sarah stood at the threshold of her living room, a radiant smile gracing her lips, her gaze fixed on the mirror before her. With each passing moment, she marveled at the subtle nuances of her reflection, the contours of her face aglow with a newfound sense of vitality and resilience. She had come to understand that the journey towards holistic well-being was not merely about shedding pounds, but rather a profound exploration of self-acceptance, resilience, and the celebration of non-scale victories that honored the intricate interplay of body, mind, and spirit.As she embarked on her journey of self-discovery, Sarah cultivated a practice of mindfulness and self-compassion that extended beyond the confines of external validation and achievement. She learned to celebrate the non-scale victories that adorned her path, recognizing the transformative power of small, incremental changes that permeated every facet of her daily life. She reveled in the newfound energy and vitality that infused her days, the sense of clarity and focus that underscored her decision-making processes, and the resilience and grace that blossomed within her with each passing day.Armed with a comprehensive understanding of the profound impact of non-scale victories, Sarah learned to cultivate a narrative of self-love and empowerment that transcended the confines of external expectations and societal constructs. She celebrated the moments of increased stamina and endurance that accompanied her regular exercise routine, the sense of accomplishment that enveloped her with each mindful and nourishing meal she prepared, and the subtle shifts in her emotional well-being and self-confidence that colored her interactions and experiences.With each non-scale victory and each moment of progress, Sarah felt the transformative power of self-acceptance infuse her life with a newfound sense of purpose and resilience. She marveled at the strength and grace that had blossomed within her, the once-familiar shadows of self-doubt and insecurity now replaced by the radiant light of self-awareness and celebration. She understood that her journey was not merely about shedding pounds, but rather about embracing a narrative of holistic well-being that honored her individuality and celebrated the boundless potential that resided within her.As she gazed at her reflection in the mirror, a sense of tranquility washed over her, a silent affirmation of the transformative power of celebrating non-scale victories and progress. She understood that each moment of self-acceptance and resilience was not merely a fleeting triumph, but rather a testament to the profound impact that self-love and empowerment had on her journey towards a life of purpose and authenticity. With a renewed sense of purpose and vitality, she stepped away from the mirror, a radiant aura of self-empowerment and resilience following in her wake, a testament to the profound impact that celebrating non-scale victories and progress had on her journey towards holistic well-being and a life of purpose and authenticity.

Chapter 22:

ADDRESSING MENTAL HEALTH AND ITS INFLUENCE ON WEIGHT LOSS

Sarah sat in quiet contemplation, the gentle embrace of her surroundings enveloping her in a sanctuary of tranquility and introspection. With each passing moment, she grappled with the profound impact of mental health on her journey towards sustainable weight management, understanding that the intricate interplay of emotions and psychological well-being played a pivotal role in shaping her relationship with food, exercise, and self-care. She had come to understand that the path to holistic well-being was not merely a physical endeavor, but rather a profound exploration of self-awareness, resilience, and the nurturing of a mind that thrived on the abundance of self-compassion and self-acceptance.As she delved into the complexities of her mental health, Sarah learned to recognize the subtle nuances of her emotional landscape, understanding that the ebb and flow of her moods and thoughts exerted a profound influence on her dietary choices, her relationship with exercise, and her capacity for self-care. She acknowledged the lingering shadows of stress and anxiety that often prompted her to seek solace in unhealthy eating habits, and the pervasive sense of self-doubt and inadequacy that hindered her sense of self-worth and resilience. With each moment of introspection and self-reflection, she began to unravel the intricate web of emotions that colored her journey towards sustainable weight management, recognizing the transformative power of cultivating a mind that thrived on the nurturing embrace of self-compassion and emotional resilience.Armed with this knowledge, Sarah endeavored to cultivate a practice of mindfulness and self-care that encompassed the dimensions of her mental and emotional well-being. She embraced the therapeutic benefits of meditation and deep breathing exercises, allowing the rhythmic cadence of her breath to ground her in the present moment and foster a sense of tranquility and equilibrium. She sought solace in the nurturing embrace of her loved ones, leaning on the wisdom and support of her community to bolster her spirits and reaffirm her commitment to self-compassion and holistic well-being.With each passing day, Sarah felt the transformative power of her emotional resilience infuse her life with a newfound sense of vitality and purpose. She marveled at the strength and grace that had blossomed within her, the once-familiar shadows of self-doubt and insecurity now replaced by the radiant light of self-acceptance and emotional equilibrium. She understood that her journey was not merely about addressing the complexities of mental health, but rather about embracing a narrative of resilience and self-empowerment that honored her individuality and celebrated the boundless potential that resided within her.As she gazed out into the world, a sense of tranquility washed over her, a silent

affirmation of the transformative power of
addressing mental health and its influence on
weight loss. She understood that each moment of
introspection and emotional resilience was not
merely a step towards self-awareness, but rather
a testament to the profound impact that self-
compassion and emotional equilibrium had on
her journey towards holistic well-being and a
life of purpose and authenticity.

Chapter 23:

MAINTENANCE AND SUSTAINING HEALTHY HABITS

Sarah stood at the crossroads of her journey, the gentle embrace of contentment and self-assurance enveloping her in a comforting embrace. With each passing moment, she marveled at the transformative power of maintenance and the sustenance of healthy habits that had guided her towards a life of sustainable well-being and resilience. She had come to understand that the pursuit of holistic wellness was not merely a fleeting endeavor, but rather a lifelong commitment to nurturing a lifestyle that honored the intricate interplay of nourishment, vitality, and self-discovery.As she delved into the intricacies of maintenance, Sarah cultivated a practice of consistency and mindfulness that extended beyond the realms of external validation and achievement. She learned to embrace the ebb and flow of her journey, understanding that the sustenance of healthy habits was not contingent on the pursuit of perfection, but rather on the cultivation of a flexible and intuitive mindset that honored the body's innate wisdom and its capacity for balance and self-regulation. She recognized the transformative power of incremental changes and small adjustments, understanding that each moment of mindfulness and self-care served as a testament to her unwavering commitment to long-term well-being and vitality.Armed with this knowledge, Sarah learned to integrate sustainable practices into every facet of her daily life, from the foods she consumed to the activities she engaged in, and the thoughts she cultivated. She embraced a diverse array of nutrient-dense foods that nourished her body from within, learning to savor each bite and to cultivate a sense of gratitude for the culinary delights that enriched her daily experiences. She fostered a regular exercise routine that brought joy and vitality into her days, understanding that movement was not merely a means to an end, but rather a celebration of the body's strength and resilience.With each passing day, Sarah felt the transformative power of her commitment to maintenance infuse her life with a newfound sense of vitality and purpose. She marveled at the resilience and grace that had blossomed within her, the once-familiar shadows of doubt and uncertainty now replaced by the radiant light of consistency and self-assurance. She understood that her journey was not merely about shedding pounds, but rather about embracing a narrative of self-care and perseverance that honored her individuality and celebrated the boundless potential that resided within her.As she turned her gaze towards the future, a sense of tranquility washed over her, a silent affirmation of the transformative power of maintenance and the sustenance of healthy habits. She understood that each moment of mindfulness and self-care was not merely an act of discipline, but rather a declaration of her unwavering commitment to self-awareness,

resilience, and the pursuit of a life that thrived
on the nurturing embrace of sustainable practices
and holistic well-being.

Chapter 24:

REACHING THE INITIAL GOAL WEIGHT AND SETTING NEW TARGETS

Sarah stood at the pinnacle of her journey, the gentle breeze of accomplishment and fulfillment enveloping her in a comforting embrace. With each passing moment, she marveled at the transformative power of resilience and determination that had guided her towards the realization of her initial goal weight. She had come to understand that the pursuit of holistic well-being was not merely about shedding pounds, but rather a profound exploration of self-discovery, perseverance, and the celebration of milestones that honored the intricate interplay of body, mind, and spirit.As she gazed at the scale before her, a radiant smile graced her lips, a testament to the unwavering commitment and discipline that had propelled her towards the realization of her initial goal weight. She reveled in the sense of accomplishment that enveloped her, understanding that the achievement was not merely a destination, but rather a reflection of the transformative power of self-awareness, resilience, and the nurturing of a lifestyle that thrived on the abundance of self-compassion and self-acceptance.Armed with this knowledge, Sarah learned to celebrate the triumphs of her journey, understanding that the realization of her initial goal weight was not the end, but rather a new beginning that beckoned her towards the exploration of new aspirations and possibilities. She recognized the transformative power of setting new targets and goals that extended beyond the confines of weight management, encompassing the dimensions of physical endurance, emotional well-being, and the cultivation of a lifestyle that honored her individuality and celebrated the boundless potential that resided within her.With each passing day, Sarah felt the transformative power of her resilience infuse her life with a newfound sense of purpose and vitality. She marveled at the strength and grace that had blossomed within her, the once-familiar shadows of self-doubt and insecurity now replaced by the radiant light of self-empowerment and self-acceptance. She understood that her journey was not merely about reaching the initial goal weight, but rather about embracing a narrative of continuous growth and self-discovery that honored her individuality and celebrated the boundless potential that resided within her.As she set her sights on new horizons, a sense of tranquility washed over her, a silent affirmation of the transformative power of setting new targets and aspirations. She understood that each moment of self-empowerment and celebration was not merely a fleeting triumph, but rather a testament to the profound impact that self-awareness and resilience had on her journey towards holistic well-being and a life of purpose and authenticity.

Chapter 25:

REFLECTING ON THE JOURNEY AND EMBRACING A NEW LIFESTYLE

Sarah sat in quiet contemplation, the echoes of her journey reverberating through the chambers of her memory, each moment a testament to the transformative power of resilience, self-awareness, and the unwavering commitment to holistic well-being. With each passing thought, she marveled at the profound impact that her experiences had on her evolution, understanding that the pursuit of a healthy lifestyle was not merely about shedding pounds, but rather a profound exploration of self-discovery, self-acceptance, and the nurturing of a lifestyle that thrived on the abundance of self-compassion and self-empowerment.As she delved into the depths of her reflections, Sarah learned to honor the myriad of experiences that had colored her journey, recognizing the transformative power of each triumph and setback, each moment of growth and self-discovery that had shaped her evolution. She reveled in the wisdom and resilience that had blossomed within her, understanding that her journey was not merely a collection of fleeting moments, but rather a tapestry of experiences that celebrated the intricate interplay of body, mind, and spirit.Armed with this newfound sense of self-awareness and gratitude, Sarah embraced a new lifestyle that honored her individuality and celebrated the boundless potential that resided within her. She integrated sustainable practices and mindful decision-making into every facet of her daily life, understanding that the pursuit of holistic well-being was not a solitary endeavor, but rather a collective commitment to nurturing a lifestyle that thrived on the nurturing embrace of self-compassion and emotional equilibrium.With each passing day, Sarah felt the transformative power of her journey infuse her life with a newfound sense of purpose and resilience. She marveled at the strength and grace that had blossomed within her, the once-familiar shadows of doubt and uncertainty now replaced by the radiant light of self-empowerment and authenticity. She understood that her journey was not merely about shedding pounds, but rather about embracing a narrative of continuous growth and self-discovery that honored her individuality and celebrated the boundless potential that resided within her.As she gazed out into the world, a sense of tranquility washed over her, a silent affirmation of the transformative power of self-reflection and the cultivation of a lifestyle that thrived on the nurturing embrace of self-compassion and authenticity. She understood that each moment of self-awareness and resilience was not merely a step towards personal growth, but rather a testament to the profound impact that self-empowerment and emotional equilibrium had on her journey towards holistic well-being and a life of purpose and fulfillment.

Summary

"Sarah's Journey: A Tale of Resilience and Self-Discovery" is an inspiring narrative that follows the protagonist, Sarah, as she grapples with the challenges of weight management and self-acceptance. Throughout the novel, Sarah confronts the complexities of fad diets, emotional eating, and societal pressures, navigating a path towards holistic well-being and self-empowerment. As she overcomes setbacks, celebrates non-scale victories, and sets new goals, Sarah's story serves as a testament to the transformative power of resilience, self-awareness, and the pursuit of a lifestyle that thrives on self-compassion and authenticity. Through her journey, readers are invited to embrace their own path towards self-discovery and holistic wellness, guided by the unwavering determination and emotional resilience that define Sarah's narrative.

www.ingramcontent.com/pod-product-compliance
Lightning Source LLC
Chambersburg PA
CBHW071600270726
48661CB00017B/261